ASIAN RECIPES

MOUTH-WATERING RECIPES TO SURPRISE YOUR FAMILY

MIKE SEAMAN

Table of Contents

Introduction

Everyone who loves to cook, loves to experiment with new dishes and new taste sensations. Chinese cuisine has become immensely popular in recent years because it offers a different range of flavours to enjoy. Most dishes are cooked on top of the stove, and many are quickly prepared and cooked so are ideal for the busy cook who wants to create an appetising and attractive dish when there is little time to spare. If you really enjoy Chinese cooking, you will probably already have a wok, and this is the perfect utensil for cooking most of the dishes in the book. If you have yet to be convinced that this style of cooking is for you, use a good frying pan or saucepan to try out the recipes. When you find how easy they are to prepare and how tasty to eat, you will almost certainly want to invest in a wok for your kitchen.

Sweet and Sour Carp

Serves 4

1 large carp or similar fish
300 g/11 oz/¬œ cup cornflour (cornstarch)
250 ml/8 fl oz/1 cup vegetable oil
30 ml/2 tbsp soy sauce
5 ml/1 tsp salt
150 g/5 oz/heaped ¬Ω cup sugar
75 ml/5 tbsp wine vinegar
15 ml/1 tbsp rice wine or dry sherry
3 spring onions (scallions), finely chopped
1 slice ginger root, finely chopped
250 ml/8 fl oz/1 cup boiling water

Clean and scale the fish and soak it for several hours in cold water. Drain and pat dry then score each side several times. Reserve 30 ml/2 tbsp of cornflour then gradually mix enough water into the remaining cornflour to make a stiff batter. Coat the fish in the batter. Heat the oil until very hot and deep-fry the fish until crisp on the outside then turn down the heat and continue to fry until the fish is tender. Meanwhile, mix together the remaining cornflour, the soy sauce, salt, sugar, wine vinegar, wine or sherry, spring onions and ginger. When the fish is cooked, transfer it to a warm serving plate. Add the sauce mixture and the water to the oil and bring to the boil, stirring well until the sauce thickens. Pour over the fish and serve immediately.

Carp with Tofu

Serves 4

1 carp
60 ml/4 tbsp groundnut (peanut) oil
225 g/8 oz tofu, cubed
2 spring onions (scallions), finely chopped
1 clove garlic, finely chopped
2 slices ginger root, finely chopped
15 ml/1 tbsp chilli sauce
30 ml/2 tbsp soy sauce
500 ml/16 fl oz/2 cups stock
30 ml/2 tbsp rice wine or dry sherry
15 ml/1 tbsp cornflour (cornstarch)
30 ml/2 tbsp water

Trim, scale and clean the fish and score 3 lines diagonally on each side. Heat the oil and fry the tofu gently until golden brown. Remove from the pan and drain well. Add the fish to the pan and fry until golden brown then remove from the pan. Pour off all but 15 ml/1 tbsp of oil then stir-fry the spring onions, garlic and ginger for 30 seconds. Add the chilli sauce, soy sauce, stock and wine and bring to the boil. Carefully add the fish to the pan with the tofu and simmer, uncovered, for about 10 minutes until the fish is cooked and the sauce reduced. Transfer the fish to a warmed serving plate and spoon the tofu on top. Blend the cornflour and water to a paste, stir it into the sauce and simmer, stirring, until the sauce thickens slightly. Spoon over the fish and serve at once.

Almond Fish Rolls

Serves 4

100 g/4 oz/1 cup almonds

450 g/1 lb cod fillets

4 slices smoked ham

1 spring onion (scallion), minced

1 slice ginger root, minced

5 ml/1 tsp cornflour (cornstarch)

5 ml/1 tsp sugar

2.5 ml/¬Ω tsp salt

15 ml/1 tbsp soy sauce

15 ml/1 tbsp rice wine or dry sherry

1 egg, lightly beaten

oil for deep-frying

1 lemon, cut into wedges

Blanch the almonds in boiling water for 5 minutes then drain and mince. Cut the fish into 9 cm/3¬Ω in squares and the ham into 5 cm/2 in squares. Mix the spring onion, ginger, cornflour, sugar, salt, soy sauce, wine or sherry and egg. Dip the fish in the mixture then lay the fish on a work surface. Coat the top with almonds then lay a slice of ham on top. Roll up the fish and tie with cook, Heat the oil and fry the fish rolls for a few minutes until golden brown. Drain on kitchen paper and serve with lemon.

Cod with Bamboo Shoots

Serves 4

4 dried Chinese mushrooms

900 g/2 lb cod fillets, cubed

30 ml/2 tbsp cornflour (cornstarch)

oil for deep-frying

30 ml/2 tbsp groundnut (peanut) oil

1 spring onion (scallion), sliced

1 slice ginger root, minced

salt

100 g/4 oz bamboo shoots, sliced

120 ml/4 fl oz/¬Ω cup fish stock

15 ml/1 tbsp soy sauce

45 ml/3 tbsp water

Soak the mushrooms in warm water for 30 minutes then drain.
Discard the stalks and slice the caps. Dust the fish with half the

cornflour. Heat the oil and deep-fry the fish until golden brown. Drain on kitchen paper and keep warm.

Meanwhile, heat the oil and fry the spring onion, ginger and salt until lightly browned. Add the bamboo shoots and stir-fry for 3 minutes. Add the stock and soy sauce, bring to the boil and simmer for 3 minutes. Mix the remaining cornflour to a paste with the water, stir into the pan and simmer, stirring, until the sauce thickens. Pour over the fish and serve at once.

Fish with Bean Sprouts

Serves 4

450 g/1 lb bean sprouts

45 ml/3 tbsp groundnut (peanut) oil

5 ml/1 tsp salt

3 slices ginger root, minced

450 g/1 lb fish fillets, sliced

4 spring onions (scallions), sliced

15 ml/1 tbsp soy sauce

60 ml/4 tbsp fish stock

10 ml/2 tsp cornflour (cornstarch)

15 ml/1 tbsp water

Blanch the bean sprouts in boiling water for 4 minutes then drain well. Heat half the oil and fry the salt and ginger for 1 minute. Add the fish and fry until lightly browned then remove it from the pan. Heat the remaining oil and fry the spring onions for 1 minute. Add the soy sauce and stock and bring to the boil. Return the fish to the pan, cover and simmer for 2 minutes until the fish is cooked. Mix the cornflour and water to a paste, stir into the pan and simmer, stirring, until the sauce clears and thickens.

Fish Fillets in Brown Sauce

Serves 4

450 g/1 lb cod fillets, thickly sliced
30 ml/2 tbsp rice wine or dry sherry
30 ml/2 tbsp soy sauce
3 spring onions (scallions), finely chopped
1 slice ginger root, finely chopped
5 ml/1 tsp salt
5 ml/1 tsp sesame oil
30 ml/2 tbsp cornflour (cornstarch)
3 eggs, beaten
90 ml/6 tbsp groundnut (peanut) oil
90 ml/6 tbsp fish stock

Place the fish fillets in a bowl. Mix together the wine or sherry, soy sauce, spring onions, ginger, salt and sesame oil, pour over the fish, cover and leave to marinate for 30 minutes. Remove the fish from the marinade and toss in the cornflour then dip in the beaten egg. Heat the oil and fry the fish until golden brown on the outside. Pour off the oil and stir in the stock and any remaining marinade. Bring to the boil and simmer gently for about 5 minutes until the fish is cooked.

Chinese Fish Cakes

Serves 4

450 g/1 lb minced (ground) cod
2 spring onions (scallions), finely chopped
1 clove garlic, crushed
5 ml/1 tsp salt
5 ml/1 tsp sugar
5 ml/1 tsp soy sauce
45 ml/3 tbsp vegetable oil
15 ml/1 tbsp cornflour (cornstarch)

Mix together the cod, spring onions, garlic, salt, sugar, soy sauce and 10 ml/2 tsp of oil. Knead together thoroughly, sprinkling with a little cornflour from time to time until the mixture is soft and elastic. Shape into 4 fish cakes. Heat the oil and fry the fish cakes for about 10 minutes until golden, pressing them flat as they cook. Serve hot or cold.

Crispy-Fried Fish

Serves 4

450 g/1 lb fish fillets, cut into strips
30 ml/2 tbsp rice wine or dry sherry
salt and freshly ground pepper
45 ml/3 tbsp cornflour (cornstarch)
1 egg white, lightly beaten
oil for deep-frying

Toss the fish in the wine or sherry and season with salt and pepper. Dust lightly with cornflour. Beat the remaining cornflour into the egg white until stiff then dip the fish in the batter. Heat the oil and deep-fry the fish strips for a few minutes until golden brown.

Deep-Fried Cod

Serves 4

900 g/2 lb cod fillets, cubed

salt and freshly ground pepper

2 eggs, beaten

100 g/4 oz/1 cup plain (all-purpose) flour

oil for deep-frying

1 lemon, cut into wedges

Season the cod with salt and pepper. Beat the eggs and flour to a batter and season with salt. Dip the fish in the batter. Heat the oil and deep-fry the fish for a few minutes until golden brown and cooked through. Drain on kitchen paper and serve with lemon wedges.

Five-Spice Fish

Serves 4

4 cod fillets

5 ml/1 tsp five-spice powder

5 ml/1 tsp salt

30 ml/2 tbsp groundnut (peanut) oil

2 cloves garlic, crushed

2.5 ml/1 in root ginger, minced

30 ml/2 tbsp rice wine or dry sherry

15 ml/1 tbsp soy sauce

few drops of sesame oil

Rub the fish with the five-spice powder and salt. Heat the oil and fry the fish until lightly browned on both sides. Remove from the pan and add the remaining ingredients. Heat through, stirring, then return the fish to the pan and reheat gently before serving.

Fragrant Fish Sticks

Serves 4

30 ml/2 tbsp rice wine or dry sherry

1 spring onion (scallion), finely chopped

2 eggs, beaten

10 ml/2 tsp curry powder

5 ml/1 tsp salt

450 g/1 lb white fish fillets, cut into strips

100 g/4 oz breadcrumbs

oil for deep-frying

Mix together the wine or sherry, spring onion, eggs, curry powder and salt. Dip the fish into the mixture so that the pieces are evenly coated then press them into the breadcrumbs. Heat the oil and deep-fry the fish for a few minutes until crisp and golden brown. Drain well and serve immediately.

Fish with Gherkins

Serves 4

4 white fish fillets

75 g/3 oz small gherkins

2 spring onions (scallions)

2 slices ginger root

30 ml/2 tbsp water

5 ml/1 tsp groundnut (peanut) oil

2.5 ml/¬Ω tsp salt

2.5 ml/¬Ω tsp rice wine or dry sherry

Place the fish on a heatproof plate and sprinkle with the remaining ingredients. Place on a rack in a steamer, cover and steam for about 15 minutes over boiling water until the fish is tender. Transfer to a warmed serving plate, discard the ginger and spring onions and serve.

Ginger-Spiced Cod

Serves 4

225 g/8 oz tomato purée (paste)

30 ml/2 tbsp rice wine or dry sherry

15 ml/1 tbsp grated ginger root

15 ml/1 tbsp chilli sauce

15 ml/1 tbsp water

15 ml/1 tbsp soy sauce

10 ml/2 tsp sugar

3 cloves garlic, crushed

100 g/4 oz/1 cup plain (all-purpose) flour

75 ml/5 tbsp cornflour (cornstarch)

175 ml/6 fl oz/¬œ cup water

1 egg white

2.5 ml/¬Ω tsp salt

oil for deep-frying

450 g/1 lb cod fillets, skinned and cubed

To make the sauce, mix together the tomato purée, wine or sherry, ginger, chilli sauce, water, soy sauce, sugar and garlic. Bring to the boil then simmer, stirring, for 4 minutes.

Beat together the flour, cornflour, water, egg white and salt until smooth. Heat the oil. Dip the fish pieces in the batter and fry for about 5 minutes until cooked through and golden brown. Drain on kitchen paper. Drain off all the oil and return the fish and sauce to the pan. Reheat gently for about 3 minutes until the fish is completely coated in sauce.

Cod with Mandarin Sauce

Serves 4

675 g/1¬Ω lb cod fillets, cut into strips

30 ml/2 tbsp cornflour (cornstarch)

60 ml/4 tbsp groundnut (peanut) oil

1 spring onion (scallion), chopped

2 cloves garlic, crushed

1 slice ginger root, minced

100 g/4 oz mushrooms, sliced

50 g/2 oz bamboo shoots, cut into strips

120 ml/4 fl oz/¬Ω cup soy sauce

30 ml/2 tbsp rice wine or dry sherry

15 ml/1 tbsp brown sugar

5 ml/1 tsp salt

250 ml/8 fl oz/1 cup chicken stock

Dip the fish in the cornflour until lightly coated. Heat the oil and fry the fish until golden brown on both sides. Remove it from the pan. Add the spring onion, garlic and ginger and stir-fry until lightly browned. Add the mushrooms and bamboo shoots and stir-fry for 2 minutes. Add the remaining ingredients and bring to the boil, stirring. Return the fish to the pan, cover and simmer for 20 minutes.

Fish with Pineapple

Serves 4

450 g/1 lb fish fillets

2 spring onions (scallions), minced

30 ml/2 tbsp soy sauce

15 ml/1 tbsp rice wine or dry sherry

2.5 ml/¬Ω tsp salt

2 eggs, lightly beaten

15 ml/1 tbsp cornflour (cornstarch)

45 ml/3 tbsp groundnut (peanut) oil

225 g/8 oz canned pineapple chunks in juice

Cut the fish into 2.5 cm/1 in strips against the grain and place in a bowl. Add the spring onions, soy sauce, wine or sherry and salt, toss well and leave to stand for 30 minutes. Drain the fish, discarding the marinade. Beat the eggs and cornflour to a batter and dip the fish in the batter to coat, draining off any excess. Heat the oil and fry the fish until lightly browned on both sides. Reduce the heat and continue to cook until tender. Meanwhile, mix 60 ml/4 tbsp of the pineapple juice with any remaining batter and the pineapple chunks. Place in a pan over a gentle heat and simmer until heated through, stirring continuously. Arrange the cooked fish on a warmed serving plate and pour over the sauce to serve.

Fish Rolls with Pork

Serves 4

450 g/1 lb fish fillets

100 g/4 oz cooked pork, minced (ground)

30 ml/2 tbsp rice wine or dry sherry

15 ml/1 tbsp sugar

oil for deep-frying

120 ml/4 fl oz/¬Ω cup fish stock

3 spring onions (scallions), minced

1 slice ginger root, minced

15 ml/1 tbsp soy sauce

15 ml/1 tbsp cornflour (cornstarch)

45 ml/3 tbsp water

Cut the fish into 9 cm/3¬Ω in squares. Mix the pork with the wine or sherry and half the sugar, spread over the fish squares, roll them up and secure with string. Heat the oil and deep-fry the fish until golden brown. Drain on kitchen paper. Meanwhile, heat the stock and add the spring onions, ginger, soy sauce and remaining sugar. Bring to the boil and simmer for 4 minutes. Mix the cornflour and water to a paste, stir into the pan and simmer, stirring, until the sauce clears and thickens. Pour over the fish and serve at once.

Fish in Rice Wine

Serves 4

400 ml/14 fl oz/1¬œ cups rice wine or dry sherry

120 ml/4 fl oz/¬Ω cup water

30 ml/2 tbsp soy sauce

5 ml/1 tsp sugar

salt and freshly ground pepper

10 ml/2 tsp cornflour (cornstarch)

15 ml/1 tbsp water

450 g/1 lb cod fillets

5 ml/1 tsp sesame oil

2 spring onions (scallions), chopped

Bring the wine, water, soy sauce, sugar, salt and pepper to the boil and boil until reduced by half. Mix the cornflour to a paste with the water, stir it into the pan and simmer, stirring, for 2 minutes. Season the fish with salt and sprinkle with sesame oil. Add to the pan and simmer very gently for about 8 minutes until cooked. Serve sprinkled with spring onions.

Quick-Fried Fish

Serves 4

450 g/1 lb cod fillets, cut into strips

salt

soy sauce

oil for deep-frying

Sprinkle the fish with salt and soy sauce and leave to stand for 10 minutes. Heat the oil and deep-fry the fish for a few minutes until lightly golden. Drain on kitchen paper and sprinkle generously with soy sauce before serving.

Sesame Seed Fish

Serves 4

450 g/1 lb fish fillets, cut into strips

1 onion, chopped

2 slices ginger root, minced

120 ml/4 fl oz/¬Ω cup rice wine or dry sherry

10 ml/2 tsp brown sugar

2.5 ml/¬Ω tsp salt

1 egg, lightly beaten

15 ml/1 tbsp cornflour (cornstarch)

45 ml/3 tbsp plain (all-purpose) flour

60 ml/6 tbsp sesame seeds

oil for deep-frying

Place the fish in a bowl. Mix together the onion, ginger, wine or sherry, sugar and salt, add to the fish and leave to marinate for 30 minutes, turning occasionally. Beat the egg, cornflour and flour to make a batter. Dip the fish in the batter then press into the sesame seeds. Heat the oil and deep-fry the fish strips for about 1 minute until golden and crispy.

Steamed Fish Balls

Serves 4

450 g/1 lb minced (ground) cod

1 egg, lightly beaten

1 slice ginger root, minced

2.5 ml/¬Ω tsp salt

pinch of freshly ground pepper

15 ml/1 tbsp cornflour (cornstarch) 15 ml/1 tbsp rice wine or dry sherry

Mix all the ingredients together well and shape into walnut-sized balls. Dust with a little flour if necessary. Arrange in a shallow ovenproof dish.

Stand the dish on a rack in a steamer, cover and steam over gently simmering water for about 10 minutes until cooked.

Marinated Sweet and Sour Fish

Serves 4

450 g/1 lb fish fillets, cut into chunks

1 onion, chopped

3 slices ginger root, minced

5 ml/1 tsp soy sauce

salt and freshly ground pepper

30 ml/2 tbsp cornflour (cornstarch)

oil for deep-frying

sweet and sour sauce

Place the fish in a bowl. Mix together the onion, ginger, soy sauce, salt and pepper, add to the fish, cover and leave to stand for 1 hour, turning occasionally. Remove the fish from the marinade and dust with cornflour. Heat the oil and deep-fry the fish until crisp and golden brown. Drain on kitchen paper and arrange on a warmed serving plate. Meanwhile, prepare the sauce and pour over the fish to serve.

Fish with Vinegar Sauce

Serves 4

450 g/1 lb fish fillets, cut into strips

salt and freshly ground pepper

1 egg white, lightly beaten

45 ml/3 tbsp cornflour (cornstarch)

15 ml/1 tbsp rice wine or dry sherry

oil for deep-frying

250 ml/8 fl oz/1 cup fish stock

15 ml/1 tbsp brown sugar

15 ml/1 tbsp wine vinegar

2 slices root ginger, minced

2 spring onions (scallions), minced

Season the fish with a little salt and pepper. Beat the egg white with 30 ml/2 tbsp of cornflour and the wine or sherry. Toss the fish in the batter until coated. Heat the oil and deep-fry the fish for a few minutes until golden brown. Drain on kitchen paper.

Meanwhile, bring the stock, sugar and wine vinegar to the boil. Add the ginger and spring onion and simmer for 3 minutes. Blend the remaining cornflour to a paste with a little water, stir it into the pan and simmer, stirring, until the sauce clears and thickens. Pour over the fish to serve.

Deep-Fried Eel

Serves 4

450 g/1 lb eel

250 ml/8 fl oz/1 cup groundnut (peanut) oil

30 ml/2 tbsp dark soy sauce

30 ml/2 tbsp rice wine or dry sherry

15 ml/1 tbsp brown sugar

dash of sesame oil

Skin the eel and cut it into chunks. Heat the oil and fry the eel until golden. Remove from the pan and drain. Pour off all but 30 ml/2 tbsp of oil. Reheat the oil and add the soy sauce, wine or sherry and sugar. Heat through then add the eel and stir-fry until the eel is well coated and almost all the liquid has evaporated. Sprinkle with sesame oil and serve.

Dry-Cooked Eel

Serves 4

5 dried Chinese mushrooms

3 spring onions (scallions)

30 ml/2 tbsp groundnut (peanut) oil

20 cloves garlic

6 slices ginger root

10 water chestnuts

900 g/2 lb eels

30 ml/2 tbsp soy sauce

15 ml/1 tbsp brown sugar

15 ml/1 tbsp rice wine or dry sherry

450 ml/¬œ pt/2 cups water

15 ml/1 tbsp cornflour (cornstarch)

45 ml/3 tbsp water

5 ml/1 tsp sesame oil

Soak the mushrooms in warm water for 30 minutes then drain and discard the stalks. Cut 1 spring onion into chunks and chop the other. Heat the oil and fry the mushrooms, spring onion chunks, garlic, ginger and chestnuts for 30 seconds. Add the eels and stir-fry for 1 minute. Add the soy sauce, sugar, wine or sherry and water, bring to the boil, cover and simmer gently for 1¬Ω hours, adding a little water during cooking if necessary. Blend the cornflour and water to a paste, stir into the pan and simmer, stirring, until the sauce thickens. Serve sprinkled with sesame oil and the chopped spring onions.

Eel with Celery

Serves 4

350 g/12 oz eel

6 stalks celery

30 ml/2 tbsp groundnut (peanut) oil

2 spring onions (scallions), chopped

1 slice ginger root, minced

30 ml/2 tbsp water

5 ml/1 tsp sugar

5 ml/1 tsp rice wine or dry sherry

5 ml/1 tsp soy sauce

freshly ground pepper

30 ml/2 tbsp chopped fresh parsley

Skin and cut the eel into strips. Cut the celery into strips. Heat the oil and fry the spring onions and ginger for 30 seconds. Add the eel and stir-fry for 30 seconds. Add the celery and stir-fry for 30 seconds. Add half the water, the sugar, wine or sherry, soy sauce and pepper. Bring to the boil and simmer for a few minutes until the celery is just tender but still crisp and the liquid has reduced. Serve sprinkled with parsley.

Haddock-Stuffed Peppers

Serves 4

225 g/8 oz haddock fillets, minced (ground)

100 g/4 oz peeled prawns, minced (ground)

1 spring onion (scallion), chopped

2.5 ml/¬Ω tsp salt

pepper

4 green peppers

45 ml/3 tbsp groundnut (peanut) oil

120 ml/4 fl oz/¬Ω cup chicken stock

10 ml/2 tsp cornflour (cornstarch)

5 ml/1 tsp soy sauce

Mix together the haddock, prawns, spring onion, salt and pepper. Cut off the stem of the peppers and lift out the centre. Stuff the peppers with the seafood mixture. Heat the oil and add the peppers and stock. Bring to the boil, cover and simmer for 15 minutes. Transfer the peppers to a warmed serving plate. Mix the cornflour, soy sauce and a little water and stir it into the pan. Bring to the boil and simmer, stirring, until the sauce clears and thickens.

Haddock in Black Bean Sauce

Serves 4

15 ml/1 tbsp groundnut (peanut) oil

2 cloves garlic, crushed

1 slice ginger root, minced

15 ml/1 tbsp black bean sauce

2 onions, cut into wedges

1 stick celery, sliced

450 g/1 lb haddock fillets

15 ml/1 tbsp soy sauce

15 ml/1 tbsp rice wine or dry sherry

250 ml/8 fl oz/1 cup chicken stock

Heat the oil and fry the garlic, ginger and black bean sauce until lightly browned. Add the onions and celery and stir-fry for 2 minutes. Add the haddock and fry for about 4 minutes each side or until the fish is cooked. Add the soy sauce, wine or sherry and chicken stock, bring to the boil, cover and simmer for 3 minutes.

Fish in Brown Sauce

Serves 4

4 haddock or similar fish

45 ml/3 tbsp groundnut (peanut) oil

2 spring onions (scallions), chopped

2 slices ginger root, chopped

5 ml/1 tsp soy sauce

2.5 ml/¬Ω tsp wine vinegar

2.5 ml/¬Ω tsp rice wine or dry sherry

2.5 ml/¬Ω tsp sugar

freshly ground pepper

2.5 ml/¬Ω tsp sesame oil

Trim the fish and cut into large chunks. Heat the oil and fry the spring onions and ginger for 30 seconds. Add the fish and fry until lightly browned on both sides. Add the soy sauce, wine vinegar, wine or sherry, sugar and pepper and simmer for 5 minutes until the sauce is thick. Serve sprinkled with sesame oil.

Five-Spice Fish

Serves 4

450 g/1 lb haddock fillets
5 ml/1 tsp five-spice powder
5 ml/1 tsp salt
30 ml/2 tbsp groundnut (peanut) oil
2 cloves garlic, crushed
2 slices ginger root, minced
30 ml/2 tbsp rice wine or dry sherry
15 ml/1 tbsp soy sauce
10 ml/2 tsp sesame oil

Rub the haddock fillets with the five-spice powder and salt. Heat the oil and fry the fish until lightly browned on both sides then remove it from the pan. Add the garlic, ginger, wine or sherry, soy sauce and sesame oil and fry for 1 minute. Return the fish to the pan and simmer gently until the fish is tender.

Haddock with Garlic

Serves 4

450 g/1 lb haddock fillets

5 ml/1 tsp salt

30 ml/2 tbsp cornflour (cornstarch)

60 ml/4 tbsp groundnut (peanut) oil

6 cloves garlic

2 slices ginger root, crushed

45 ml/3 tbsp water

30 ml/2 tbsp soy sauce

15 ml/1 tbsp yellow bean sauce

15 ml/1 tbsp rice wine or dry sherry

15 ml/1 tbsp brown sugar

Sprinkle the haddock with salt and dust with cornflour. Heat the oil and fry the fish until golden brown on both sides then remove it from the pan. Add the garlic and ginger and fry for 1 minute. Add the remaining ingredients, bring to the boil, cover and simmer for 5 minutes. Return the fish to the pan, cover and simmer until tender.

Hot-Spiced Fish

Serves 4

450 g/1 lb haddock fillets, diced

juice of 1 lemon

30 ml/2 tbsp soy sauce

30 ml/2 tbsp oyster sauce

15 ml/1 tbsp grated lemon rind

pinch of ground ginger

salt and pepper

2 egg whites

45 ml/3 tbsp cornflour (cornstarch)

6 dried Chinese mushrooms

oil for deep-frying

5 spring onions (scallions), cut into strips

1 stick celery, cut into strips

100 g/4 oz bamboo shoots, cut into strips

250 ml/8 fl oz/1 cup chicken stock

5 ml/1 tsp five-spice powder

Put the fish in a bowl and sprinkle with lemon juice. Mix together the soy sauce, oyster sauce, lemon rind, ginger, salt, pepper, egg whites and all but 5 ml/1 tsp of the cornflour. Leave to marinate for 2 hours, stirring occasionally. Soak the mushrooms in warm water for 30 minutes then drain. Discard the stalks and slice the caps. Heat the oil and fry the fish for a few minutes until golden. Remove from the pan. Add the vegetables and fry until tender but still crisp. Pour off the oil. Mix the chicken stock with the remaining cornflour, add it to the vegetables and bring to the boil. Return the fish to the pan, season with five-spice powder and heat through before serving.

Ginger Haddock with Pak Soi

Serves 4

450 g/1 lb haddock fillet

salt and pepper

225 g/8 oz pak soi

30 ml/2 tbsp groundnut (peanut) oil

1 slice ginger root, chopped

1 onion, chopped

2 dried red chilli peppers

5 ml/1 tsp honey

10 ml/2 tsp tomato ketchup (catsup)

10 ml/2 tsp malt vinegar

30 ml/2 tbsp dry white wine

10 ml/2 tsp soy sauce

10 ml/2 tsp fish sauce

10 ml/2 tsp oyster sauce

5 ml/1 tsp shrimp paste

Skin the haddock then cut into 2 cm/ ¬æ in pieces. Sprinkle with salt and pepper. Cut the cabbage into small pieces. Heat the oil and fry the ginger and onion for 1 minute. Add the cabbage and chilli peppers and fry for 30 seconds. Add the honey, tomato ketchup, vinegar and wine. Add the haddock and simmer for 2 minutes. Stir in the soy, fish and oyster sauces and the shrimp paste and simmer gently until the haddock is cooked.

Haddock Plaits

Serves 4

450 g/1 lb haddock fillets, skinned

salt

5 ml/1 tsp five-spice powder

juice of 2 lemons

5 ml/1 tsp aniseed, ground

5 ml/1 tsp freshly ground pepper

30 ml/2 tbsp soy sauce

30 ml/2 tbsp oyster sauce

15 ml/1 tbsp honey

60 ml/4 tbsp chopped chives

8,Äì10 spinach leaves

45 ml/3 tbsp wine vinegar

Cut the fish into long thin strips and shape into plaits, sprinkle with salt, five-spice powder and lemon juice and transfer to a bowl. Mix together the aniseed, pepper, soy sauce, oyster sauce, honey and chives, pour over the fish and leave to marinate for at least 30 minutes. Line the steam basket with the spinach leaves, place the plaits on top, cover and steam over gently boiling water with the vinegar for about 25 minutes.

Steamed Fish Roulades

Serves 4

450 g/1 lb haddock fillets, skinned and diced

juice of 1 lemon

30 ml/2 tbsp soy sauce

30 ml/2 tbsp oyster sauce

30 ml/2 tbsp plum sauce

5 ml/1 tsp rice wine or dry sherry

salt and pepper

6 dried Chinese mushrooms

100 g/4 oz bean sprouts

100 g/4 oz green peas

50 g/2 oz/¬Ω cup walnuts, chopped

1 egg, beaten

30 ml/2 tbsp cornflour (cornstarch)

225 g/8 oz Chinese cabbage, blanched

Put the fish in a bowl. Mix together the lemon juice, soy, oyster and plum sauces, wine or sherry and salt and pepper. Pour over the fish and leave to marinate for 30 minutes. Add the vegetables, nuts, egg and cornflour and mix together well. Lay 3 Chinese leaves on top of each other, spoon on some of the fish mixture and roll up. Continue until all the ingredients have been used up. Place the rolls in a steam basket, cover and cook over gently simmering water for 30 minutes.

Halibut with Tomato Sauce

Serves 4

450 g/1 lb halibut fillets

salt

15 ml/1 tbsp black bean sauce

1 clove garlic, crushed

2 spring onions (scallions), chopped

2 slices ginger root, minced

15 ml/1 tbsp rice wine or dry sherry

15 ml/1 tbsp soy sauce

200 g/7 oz canned tomatoes, drained

30 ml/2 tbsp groundnut (peanut) oil

Sprinkle the halibut generously with salt and leave to stand for 1 hour. Rinse off the salt and pat dry. Place the fish in an ovenproof bowl and sprinkle with the black bean sauce, garlic, spring onions, ginger, wine or sherry, soy sauce and tomatoes. Place the bowl on a rack in a steamer, cover and steam for 20 minutes over boiling water until the fish is cooked. Heat the oil until almost smoking and sprinkle over the fish before serving.

Monkfish with Broccoli

Serves 4

450 g/1 lb monkfish tail, cubed

salt and pepper

45 ml/3 tbsp groundnut (peanut) oil

50 g/2 oz mushrooms, sliced

1 small carrot, cut into strips

1 clove garlic, crushed

2 slices ginger root, minced

45 ml/3 tbsp water

275 g/10 oz broccoli florets

5 ml/1 tsp sugar

5 ml/1 tsp cornflour (cornstarch)

45 ml/3 tbsp water

Season the monkfish well with salt and pepper. Heat 30 ml/2 tbsp of oil and fry the monkfish, mushrooms, carrot, garlic and ginger until lightly browned. Add the water and continue to simmer, uncovered, over a low heat. Meanwhile, blanch the broccoli in boiling water until just tender then drain well. Heat the remaining oil and stir-fry the broccoli and sugar with a pinch of salt until the broccoli is well coated in the oil. Arrange round a warmed serving plate. Mix the cornflour and water to a paste, stir into the fish and simmer, stirring, until the sauce thickens. Pour over the broccoli and serve at once.

Serves 4

1 red mullet

oil for deep-frying

30 ml/2 tbsp groundnut (peanut) oil

2 spring onions (scallions), sliced

2 slices ginger root, shredded

1 red chilli pepper, shredded

250 ml/8 fl oz/1 cup fish stock

15 ml/1 tbsp thick soy sauce

15 ml/1 tbsp freshly ground white

pepper

15 ml/1 tbsp rice wine or dry sherry

Trim the fish and score it diagonally on each side. Heat the oil and deep-fry the fish until half cooked. Remove from the oil and drain well. Heat the oil and fry the spring onions, ginger and chilli pepper for 1 minute. Add the remaining ingredients, stir together well and bring to the boil. Add the fish and simmer gently, uncovered, until the fish is cooked and the liquid has almost evaporated.

West Lake Fish

Serves 4

1 mullet

30 ml/2 tbsp groundnut (peanut) oil

4 spring onions (scallions), shredded

1 red chilli pepper, chopped

4 slices ginger root, shredded

45 ml/3 tbsp brown sugar

30 ml/2 tbsp red wine vinegar

30 ml/2 tbsp water

30 ml/2 tbsp soy sauce

freshly ground pepper

Clean and trim the fish and make 2 or 3 diagonal cuts on each side. Heat the oil and stir-fry half the spring onions, the chilli pepper and ginger for 30 seconds. Add the fish and fry until lightly browned on both sides. Add the sugar, wine vinegar, water, soy sauce and pepper, bring to the boil, cover and simmer for about 20 minutes until the fish is cooked and the sauce has reduced. Serve garnished with the remaining spring onions.

Fried Plaice

Serves 4

4 plaice fillets
salt and freshly ground pepper
30 ml/2 tbsp groundnut (peanut) oil
1 slice ginger root, minced
1 clove garlic, crushed
lettuce leaves

Season the plaice generously with salt and pepper. Heat the oil and fry the ginger and garlic for 20 seconds. Add the fish and fry until cooked through and golden brown. Drain well and serve on a bed of lettuce.

Steamed Plaice with Chinese Mushrooms

Serves 4

4 dried Chinese mushrooms

450 g/1 lb plaice fillets, cubed

1 clove garlic, crushed

1 slice ginger root, minced

15 ml/1 tbsp soy sauce

15 ml/1 tbsp rice wine or dry sherry

5 ml/1 tsp brown sugar

350 g/12 oz cooked long-grain rice

Soak the mushrooms in warm water for 30 minutes then drain. Discard the stems and chop the caps. Mix with the plaice, garlic, ginger, soy sauce, wine or sherry and sugar, cover and leave to marinate for 1 hour. Place the rice in a steamer and arrange the fish on top. Steam for about 30 minutes until the fish is cooked.

Plaice with Garlic

Serves 4

350 g/12 oz plaice fillets

salt

45 ml/3 tbsp cornflour (cornstarch)

1 egg, beaten

60 ml/4 tbsp groundnut (peanut) oil

3 cloves garlic, chopped

4 spring onions (scallions), chopped

15 ml/1 tbsp rice wine or dry sherry

5 ml/1 tsp sesame oil

Skin the plaice and cut it into strips. Sprinkle with salt and leave to stand for 20 minutes. Dust the fish with cornflour then dip in the egg. Heat the oil and fry the fish strips for about 4 minutes until golden brown. Remove from the pan and drain on kitchen paper. Pour off all but 5 ml/1 tsp of oil from the pan and add the remaining ingredients. Bring to the boil, stirring, then simmer for 3 minutes. Pour over the fish and serve immediately.

Plaice with Pineapple Sauce

Serves 4

450 g/1 lb plaice fillets

5 ml/1 tsp salt

30 ml/2 tbsp soy sauce

200 g/7 oz canned pineapple chunks

2 eggs, beaten

100 g/4 oz/¬Ω cup cornflour (cornstarch)

oil for deep-frying

30 ml/2 tbsp water

5 ml/1 tsp sesame oil

Cut the plaice into strips and place in a bowl. Sprinkle with salt, soy sauce and 30 ml/2 tbsp of the pineapple juice and leave to stand for 10 minutes. Beat the eggs with 45 ml/3 tbsp of cornflour to a batter and dip the fish in the batter. Heat the oil and deep-fry the fish until golden brown. Drain on kitchen pepper. Put the remaining pineapple juice in a small saucepan. Blend 30 ml/2 tbsp of cornflour with the water and stir it into the pan. Bring to the boil and simmer, stirring, until thickened. Add half the pineapple pieces and heat through. Just before serving, stir in the sesame oil. Arrange the cooked fish on a warmed serving plate and garnish with the reserved pineapple. Pour over the hot sauce and serve at once.

Salmon with Tofu

Serves 4

120 ml/4 fl oz/¬Ω cup groundnut (peanut) oil

450 g/1 lb tofu, cubed

2.5 ml/¬Ω tsp sesame oil

100 g/4 oz salmon fillet, chopped

dash of chilli sauce

250 ml/8 fl oz/1 cup fish stock

15 ml/1 tbsp cornflour (cornstarch)

45 ml/3 tbsp water

2 spring onions (scallions), chopped

Heat the oil and fry the tofu until lightly browned. Remove from the pan. Reheat the oil and sesame oil and fry the salmon and chilli sauce for 1 minute. Add the stock, bring to the boil, then return the tofu to the pan. Simmer gently, uncovered, until the ingredients are cooked through and the liquid has reduced. Blend the cornflour and water to a paste. Stir in a little at a time and simmer, stirring, until the mixture thickens. You may not need all the cornflour paste if you have allowed the liquid to reduce. Transfer to a warmed serving plate and sprinkle with the spring onions.

Deep-Fried Marinated Fish

Serves 4

450 g/1 lb sprats or other small fish, cleaned

3 slices ginger root, minced

120 ml/4 fl oz/¬Ω cup soy sauce

15 ml/1 tbsp rice wine or dry sherry

1 clove star anise

oil for deep-frying

15 ml/1 tbsp sesame oil

Place the fish in a bowl. Mix together the ginger, soy sauce, wine or sherry and anise, pour over the fish and leave to stand for 1 hour, turning occasionally. Drain the fish, discarding the marinade. Heat the oil and fry the fish in batches until crispy and golden brown. Drain on kitchen paper and serve sprinkled with sesame oil.

Trout with Carrots

Serves 4

15 ml/1 tbsp groundnut (peanut) oil

1 clove garlic, crushed

1 slice ginger root, minced

4 trout

2 carrots, cut into strips

25 g/1 oz bamboo shoots, cut into strips

25 g/1 oz water chestnuts, cut into strips

15 ml/1 tbsp soy sauce

15 ml/1 tbsp rice wine or dry sherry

Heat the oil and fry the garlic and ginger until lightly browned. Add the fish, cover and fry until the fish turns opaque. Add the carrots, bamboo shoots, chestnuts, soy sauce and wine or sherry, stir carefully, cover and simmer for about 5 minutes.

Deep-Fried Trout

Serves 4

4 trout, cleaned and scaled

2 eggs, beaten

50 g/2 oz/¬Ω cup plain (all-purpose) flour

oil for deep-frying

1 lemon, cut into wedges

Slash the fish diagonally a few times on each side. Dip in the beaten eggs then toss in the flour to coat completely. Shake off any excess. Heat the oil and deep-fry the fish for about 10 to 15 minutes until cooked. Drain on kitchen paper and serve with lemon.

Trout with Lemon Sauce

Serves 4

450 ml/¬œ pt/2 cups chicken stock

5 cm/2 in square piece lemon rind

150 ml/¬° pt/generous ¬Ω cup lemon juice

90 ml/6 tbsp brown sugar

2 slices ginger root, cut into strips

30 ml/2 tbsp cornflour (cornstarch)

4 trout

375 g/12 oz/3 cups plain (all-purpose) flour

175 ml/6 fl oz/¬œ cup water

oil for deep-frying

2 egg whites

8 spring onions (scallions), thinly sliced

To make the sauce, mix together the stock, lemon rind and juice, sugar and for 5 minutes. Remove from the heat, strain and return to the pan. Mix the cornflour with a little water then stir it into the pan. Simmer for 5 minutes, stirring frequently. Remove from the heat and keep the sauce warm.

Lightly coat the fish on both sides with a little of the flour. Beat the remaining flour with the water and 10 ml/2 tsp of oil until smooth. Beat the egg whites until stiff but not dry and fold them into the batter. Heat the remaining oil. Dip the fish in the batter to coat it completely. Cook the fish for about 10 minutes, turning once, until cooked through and golden. Drain on kitchen paper. Arrange the fish on a warmed serving plate. Stir the spring onions into the warm sauce, pour over the fish and serve immediately.

Chinese Tuna

Serves 4

30 ml/2 tbsp groundnut (peanut) oil

1 onion, chopped

200 g/7 oz canned tuna, drained and flaked

2 stalks celery, chopped

100 g/4 oz mushrooms, chopped

1 green pepper, chopped

250 ml/8 fl oz/1 cup stock

30 ml/2 tbsp soy sauce

100 g/4 oz fine egg noodles

salt

15 ml/1 tbsp cornflour (cornstarch)

45 ml/3 tbsp water

Heat the oil and fry the onion until softened. Add the tuna and stir until well coated with oil. Add the celery, mushrooms and pepper and stir-fry for 2 minutes. Add the stock and soy sauce, bring to the boil, cover and simmer for 15 minutes. Meanwhile, cook the noodles in boiling salt water for about 5 minutes until just tender then drain well and arrange on a warmed serving plate. Mix the cornflour and water, stir the mixture into the tuna sauce and simmer, stirring, until the sauce clears and thickens.

Marinated Fish Steaks

Serves 4

4 whiting or haddock steaks
2 cloves garlic, crushed
2 slices ginger root, crushed
3 spring onions (scallions), chopped
15 ml/1 tbsp rice wine or dry sherry
15 ml/1 tbsp wine vinegar
salt and freshly ground pepper
45 ml/3 tbsp groundnut (peanut) oil

Place the fish in a bowl. Mix the garlic, ginger, spring onions, wine or sherry, wine vinegar, salt and pepper, pour over the fish, cover and leave to marinate for several hours. Remove the fish from the marinade. Heat the oil and fry the fish until browned on both sides then remove from the pan. Add the marinade to the pan, bring to the boil then return the fish to the pan and simmer gently until cooked through.

Prawns with Almonds

Serves 4

100 g/4 oz almonds

225 g/8 oz large unpeeled prawns

2 slices ginger root, minced

15 ml/1 tbsp cornflour (cornstarch)

2.5 ml/¬Ω tsp salt

30 ml/2 tbsp groundnut (peanut) oil

2 cloves garlic

2 stalks celery, chopped

5 ml/1 tsp soy sauce

5 ml/1 tsp rice wine or dry sherry

30 ml/2 tbsp water

Toast the almonds in a dry pan until lightly browned then put to one side. Peel the prawns, leaving on the tails, and cut in half lengthways to the tail. Mix with the ginger, cornflour and salt. Heat the oil and fry the garlic until lightly browned then discard the garlic. Add the celery, soy sauce, wine or sherry and water to the pan and bring to the boil. Add the prawns and stir-fry until heated through. Serve sprinkled with toasted almonds.

Anise Prawns

Serves 4

45 ml/3 tbsp groundnut (peanut) oil

15 ml/1 tbsp soy sauce

5 ml/1 tsp sugar

120 ml/4 fl oz/¬Ω cup fish stock

pinch of ground anise

450 g/1 lb peeled prawns

Heat the oil, add the soy sauce, sugar, stock and anise and bring to the boil. Add the prawns and simmer for a few minutes until heated through and flavoured.

Prawns with Asparagus

Serves 4

450 g/1 lb asparagus, cut into chunks

45 ml/3 tbsp groundnut (peanut) oil

2 slices ginger root, minced

15 ml/1 tbsp soy sauce

15 ml/1 tbsp rice wine or dry sherry

5 ml/1 tsp sugar

2.5 ml/¬Ω tsp salt

225 g/8 oz peeled prawns

Blanch the asparagus in boiling water for 2 minutes then drain well. Heat the oil and fry the ginger for a few seconds. Add the asparagus and stir until well coated with oil. Add the soy sauce, wine or sherry, sugar and salt and heat through. Add the prawns and stir over a low heat until the asparagus is tender.

Prawns with Bacon

Serves 4

450 g/1 lb large unpeeled prawns

100 g/4 oz bacon

1 egg, lightly beaten

2.5 ml/¬Ω tsp salt

15 ml/1 tbsp soy sauce

50 g/2 oz/¬Ω cup cornflour (cornstarch)

oil for deep-frying

Peel the prawns, leaving the tails intact. Cut in half lengthways to the tail. Cut the bacon into small squares. Press a piece of bacon in the centre of each prawn and press the two halves together. Beat the egg with the salt and soy sauce. Dip the prawns in the egg then dust with cornflour. Heat the oil and deep-fry the prawns until crispy and golden.

Prawn Balls

Serves 4

3 dried Chinese mushrooms
450 g/1 lb prawns, finely minced
6 water chestnuts, finely minced
1 spring onion (scallion), finely minced
1 slice ginger root, finely minced
salt and freshly ground pepper
2 eggs, beaten
15 ml/1 tbsp cornflour (cornstarch)
50 g/2 oz/¬Ω cup plain (all-purpose) flour
groundnut (peanut) oil for deep-frying

Soak the mushrooms in warm water for 30 minutes then drain. Discard the stems and finely chop the caps. Mix with the prawns, water chestnuts, spring onion and ginger and season with salt and pepper. Mix in 1 egg and 5 ml/1 tsp cornflour roll into balls about the size of a heaped teaspoon.

Beat together the remaining egg, cornflour and flour and add enough water to make a thick, smooth batter. Roll the balls in the batter. Heat the oil and deep-fry for a few minutes until light golden brown.

Barbecued Prawns

Serves 4

450 g/1 lb large peeled prawns
100 g/4 oz bacon
225 g/8 oz chicken livers, sliced
1 clove garlic, crushed
2 slices ginger root, minced
30 ml/2 tbsp sugar
120 ml/4 fl oz/¬Ω cup soy sauce
salt and freshly ground pepper

Cut the prawns lengthways down the back without cutting right through and flatten them slightly. Cut the bacon into chunks and place in a bowl with the prawns and chicken livers. Mix together the remaining ingredients, pour over the prawns and leave to stand for 30 minutes. Thread the prawns, bacon and livers oh to skewers and grill or barbecue for about 5 minutes, turning frequently, until cooked through, basting occasionally with the marinade.

Prawns with Bamboo Shoots

Serves 4

60 ml/4 tbsp groundnut (peanut) oil

1 clove garlic, minced

1 slice ginger root, minced

450 g/1 lb peeled prawns

30 ml/2 tbsp rice wine or dry sherry

225 g/8 oz bamboo shoots

30 ml/2 tbsp soy sauce

15 ml/1 tbsp cornflour (cornstarch)

45 ml/3 tbsp water

Heat the oil and fry the garlic and ginger until lightly browned. Add the prawns and stir-fry for 1 minute. Add the wine or sherry and stir together well. Add the bamboo shoots and stir-fry for 5 minutes. Add the remaining ingredients and stir-fry for 2 minutes.

Prawns with Bean Sprouts

Serves 4

4 dried Chinese mushrooms
30 ml/2 tbsp groundnut (peanut) oil
1 clove garlic, crushed
225 g/8 oz peeled prawns
15 ml/1 tbsp rice wine or dry sherry
450 g/1 lb bean sprouts
120 ml/4 fl oz/¬Ω cup chicken stock
15 ml/1 tbsp soy sauce
15 ml/1 tbsp cornflour (cornstarch)
salt and freshly ground pepper
2 spring onion (scallions), chopped

Soak the mushrooms in warm water for 30 minutes then drain. Discard the stems and slice the caps. Heat the oil and fry the garlic until lightly browned. Add the prawns and stir-fry for 1 minute. Add the wine or sherry and fry for 1 minute. Stir in the mushrooms and bean sprouts. Mix together the stock, soy sauce and cornflour and stir it into the pan. Bring to the boil then simmer, stirring, until the sauce clears and thickens. Season to taste with salt and pepper. Serve sprinkled with spring onions.

Prawns with Black Bean Sauce

Serves 4

30 ml/2 tbsp groundnut (peanut) oil

5 ml/1 tsp salt

1 clove garlic, crushed

45 ml/3 tbsp black bean sauce

1 green pepper, chopped

1 onion, chopped

120 ml/4 fl oz/¬Ω cup fish stock

5 ml/1 tsp sugar

15 ml/1 tbsp soy sauce

225 g/8 oz peeled prawns

15 ml/1 tbsp cornflour (cornstarch)

45 ml/3 tbsp water

Heat the oil and stir-fry the salt, garlic and black bean sauce for 2 minutes. Add the pepper and onion and stir-fry for 2 minutes. Add the stock, sugar and soy sauce and bring to the boil. Add the prawns and simmer for 2 minutes. Mix the cornflour and water to a paste, add it to the pan and simmer, stirring, until the sauce clears and thickens.

Prawns with Celery

Serves 4

45 ml/3 tbsp groundnut (peanut) oil

3 slices ginger root, minced

450 g/1 lb peeled prawns

5 ml/1 tsp salt

15 ml/1 tbsp sherry

4 stalks celery, chopped

100 g/4 oz almonds, chopped

Heat half the oil and fry the ginger until lightly browned. Add the prawns, salt and sherry and stir-fry until well coated in oil then remove from the pan. Heat the remaining oil and stir-fry the celery and almonds for a few minutes until the celery is just tender but still crisp. Return the prawns to the pan, mix well and heat through before serving.

Stir-Fried Prawns with Chicken

Serves 4

30 ml/2 tbsp groundnut (peanut) oil

2 cloves garlic, crushed

225 g/8 oz cooked chicken, thinly sliced

100 g/4 oz bamboo shoots, sliced

100 g/4 oz mushrooms, sliced

75 ml/5 tbsp fish stock

225 g/8 oz peeled prawns

225 g/8 oz mangetout (snow peas)

15 ml/1 tbsp cornflour (cornstarch)

45 ml/3 tbsp water

Heat the oil and fry the garlic until lightly browned. Add the chicken, bamboo shoots and mushrooms and stir-fry until well coated in oil. Add the stock and bring to the boil. Add the prawns and mangetout, cover and simmer for 5 minutes. Mix the cornflour and water to a paste, stir into the pan and simmer, stirring, until the sauce clears and thickens. Serve at once.

Chilli Prawns

Serves 4

450 g/1 lb peeled prawns

1 egg white

10 ml/2 tsp cornflour (cornstarch)

5 ml/1 tsp salt

60 ml/4 tbsp groundnut (peanut) oil

25 g/1 oz dried red chilli peppers, trimmed

1 clove garlic, crushed

5 ml/1 tsp freshly ground pepper

15 ml/1 tbsp soy sauce

5 ml/1 tsp rice wine or dry sherry

2.5 ml/¬Ω tsp sugar

2.5 ml/¬Ω tsp wine vinegar

2.5 ml/¬Ω tsp sesame oil

Place the prawns in a bowl with the egg white, cornflour and salt and leave to marinate for 30 minutes. Heat the oil and fry the chilli peppers, garlic and pepper for 1 minute. Add the prawns and remaining ingredients and stir-fry for a few minutes until the prawns are heated through and the ingredients well mixed.

Prawn Chop Suey

Serves 4

60 ml/4 tbsp groundnut (peanut) oil

2 spring onions (scallions), chopped

2 cloves garlic, crushed

1 slice ginger root, chopped

225 g/8 oz peeled prawns

100 g/4 oz frozen peas

100 g/4 oz button mushrooms, halved

30 ml/2 tbsp soy sauce

15 ml/1 tbsp rice wine or dry sherry

5 ml/1 tsp sugar

5 ml/1 tsp salt

15 ml/1 tbsp cornflour (cornstarch)

Heat 45 ml/3 tbsp of oil and fry the spring onions, garlic and ginger until lightly browned. Add the prawns and stir-fry for 1 minute. Remove from the pan. Heat the remaining oil and stir-fry the peas and mushrooms for 3 minutes. Add the prawns, soy sauce, wine or sherry, sugar and salt and stir-fry for 2 minutes. Mix the cornflour with a little water, stir it into the pan and simmer, stirring, until the sauce clears and thickens.

Prawn Chow Mein

Serves 4

450 g/1 lb peeled prawns
15 ml/1 tbsp cornflour (cornstarch)
15 ml/1 tbsp soy sauce
15 ml/1 tbsp rice wine or dry sherry
4 dried Chinese mushrooms
30 ml/2 tbsp groundnut (peanut) oil
5 ml/1 tsp salt
1 slice ginger root, minced
100 g/4 oz Chinese cabbage, sliced
100 g/4 oz bamboo shoots, sliced
Soft-Fried Noodles

Mix the prawns with the cornflour, soy sauce and wine or sherry and leave to stand, stirring occasionally. Soak the mushrooms in warm water for 30 minutes then drain. Discard the stalks and slice the caps. Heat the oil and fry the salt and ginger for 1 minute. Add the cabbage and bamboo shoots and stir until coated with oil. Cover and simmer for 2 minutes. Stir in the prawns and marinade and stir-fry for 3 minutes. Stir in the drained noodles and heat through before serving.

Prawns with Courgettes and Lychees

Serves 4

12 king prawns

salt and pepper

10 ml/2 tsp soy sauce

10 ml/2 tsp cornflour (cornstarch)

15 ml/1 tbsp groundnut (peanut) oil

4 cloves garlic, crushed

2 red chilli peppers, chopped

225 g/8 oz courgettes (zucchini), diced

2 spring onions (scallions), chopped

12 lychees, stoned

120 ml/4 fl oz/¬Ω cup coconut cream

10 ml/2 tsp mild curry powder

5 ml/1 tsp fish sauce

Peel the prawns, leaving on the tails. Sprinkle with salt, pepper and soy sauce then coat with cornflour. Heat the oil and fry the garlic, chilli peppers and prawns for 1 minute. Add the courgettes, spring onions and lychees and stir-fry for 1 minute. Remove from the pan. Pour the coconut cream into the pan, bring to the boil and simmer for 2 minutes until thick. Stir in the curry powder and fish sauce and season with salt and pepper. Return the prawns and vegetables to the sauce to heat through before serving.

Prawns with Crab

Serves 4

45 ml/3 tbsp groundnut (peanut) oil
3 spring onions (scallions), chopped
1 sliced ginger root, minced
225 g/8 oz crab meat
15 ml/1 tbsp rice wine or dry sherry
30 ml/2 tbsp chicken or fish stock
15 ml/1 tbsp soy sauce
5 ml/1 tsp brown sugar
5 ml/1 tsp wine vinegar
freshly ground pepper
10 ml/2 tsp cornflour (cornstarch)
225 g/8 oz peeled prawns

Heat 30 ml/2 tbsp of oil and fry the spring onions and ginger until lightly browned. Add the crab meat and stir-fry for 2 minutes. Add the wine or sherry, stock, soy sauce, sugar and vinegar and season to taste with pepper. Stir-fry for 3 minutes. Mix the cornflour with a little water and stir it into the sauce. Simmer, stirring, until the sauce thickens. Meanwhile, heat the remaining oil in a separate pan and stir-fry the prawns for a few minutes until heated through. Arrange the crab mixture on a warmed serving plate and top with the prawns.

Prawns with Cucumber

Serves 4

225 g/8 oz peeled prawns
salt and freshly ground pepper
15 ml/1 tbsp cornflour (cornstarch)
1 cucumber
45 ml/3 tbsp groundnut (peanut) oil
2 cloves garlic, crushed
1 onion, finely chopped
15 ml/1 tbsp rice wine or dry sherry
2 slices ginger root, minced

Season the prawns with salt and pepper and toss with the cornflour. Peel and seed the cucumber and cut it into thick slices. Heat half the oil and fry the garlic and onion until lightly browned. Add the prawns and sherry and stir-fry for 2 minutes then remove the ingredients from the pan. Heat the remaining oil and fry the ginger for 1 minute. Add the cucumber and stir-fry for 2 minutes. Return the prawn mixture to the pan and stir-fry until well mixed and heated through.

Prawn Curry

Serves 4

45 ml/3 tbsp groundnut (peanut) oil

4 spring onions (scallions), sliced

30 ml/2 tbsp curry powder

2.5 ml/¬Ω tsp salt

120 ml/4 fl oz/¬Ω cup chicken stock

450 g/1 lb peeled prawns

Heat the oil and fry the spring onions for 30 seconds. Add the curry powder and salt and stir-fry for 1 minute. Add the stock, bring to the boil and simmer, stirring, for 2 minutes. Add the prawns and heat through gently.

Prawn and Mushroom Curry

Serves 4

5 ml/1 tsp soy sauce

5 ml/1 tsp rice wine or dry sherry

225 g/8 oz peeled prawns

30 ml/2 tbsp groundnut (peanut) oil

2 cloves garlic, crushed

1 slice ginger root, finely chopped

1 onion, cut into wedges

100 g/4 oz button mushrooms

100 g/4 oz fresh or frozen peas

15 ml/1 tbsp curry powder

15 ml/1 tbsp cornflour (cornstarch)

150 ml/¬° pt/generous ¬Ω cup chicken stock

Mix together the soy sauce, wine or sherry and prawns. Heat the oil with the garlic and ginger and fry until lightly browned. Add the onion, mushrooms and peas and stir-fry for 2 minutes. Add the curry powder and cornflour and stir-fry for 2 minutes. Gradually stir in the stock, bring to the boil, cover and simmer for 5 minutes, stirring occasionally. Add the prawns and marinade, cover and simmer for 2 minutes.

Deep-Fried Prawns

Serves 4

450 g/1 lb peeled prawns

30 ml/2 tbsp rice wine or dry sherry

5 ml/1 tsp salt

oil for deep-frying

soy sauce

Toss the prawns in the wine or sherry and sprinkle with salt. Leave to stand for 15 minutes then drain and pat dry. Heat the oil and deep-fry the prawns for a few seconds until crisp. Serve sprinkled with soy sauce.

Deep-Fried Battered Prawns

Serves 4

50 g/2 oz/¬Ω cup plain (all-purpose) flour

2.5 ml/¬Ω tsp salt

1 egg, lightly beaten

30 ml/2 tbsp water

450 g/1 lb peeled prawns

oil for deep-frying

Beat the flour, salt, egg and water to a batter, adding a little more water if necessary. Mix with the prawns until well coated. Heat the oil and deep-fry the prawns for a few minutes until crispy and golden.

Prawn Dumplings with Tomato Sauce

Serves 4

900 g/2 lb peeled prawns

450 g/1 lb minced (ground) cod

4 eggs, beaten

50 g/2 oz/¬Ω cup cornflour (cornstarch)

2 cloves garlic, crushed

30 ml/2 tbsp soy sauce

15 ml/1 tbsp sugar

15 ml/1 tbsp groundnut (peanut) oil

For the sauce:

30 ml/2 tbsp groundnut (peanut) oil

100 g/4 oz spring onions (scallions), chopped

100 g/4 oz mushrooms, chopped

100 g/4 oz ham, chopped

2 stalks celery, chopped

200 g/7 oz tomatoes, skinned and chopped

300 ml/¬Ω pt/1¬° cups water

salt and freshly ground pepper

15 ml/1 tbsp cornflour (cornstarch)

Finely chop the prawns and mix with the cod. Stir in the eggs, cornflour, garlic, soy sauce, sugar and oil. Bring a large saucepan of water to the boil and drop spoonfuls of the mixture into the saucepan. Return to the boil and simmer for a few minutes until the dumplings float to the surface. Drain well. To make the sauce, heat the oil and fry the spring onions until soft but not browned. Add the mushrooms and fry for 1 minute then add the ham, celery and tomatoes and fry for 1 minute. Add the water, bring to the boil and season with salt and pepper. Cover and simmer for 10 minutes, stirring occasionally. Mix the cornflour with a little water and stir it into the sauce. Simmer for a few minutes, stirring, until the sauce clears and thickens. Serve with the dumplings.

Prawn and Egg Cups

Serves 4

15 ml/1 tbsp sesame oil
8 peeled king prawns
1 red chilli pepper, chopped
2 spring onions (scallions), chopped
30 ml/2 tbsp chopped abalone (optional)
8 eggs
15 ml/1 tbsp soy sauce
salt and freshly ground pepper
few sprigs of flat-leaved parsley

Use the sesame oil to grease 8 ramekin dishes. Place one prawn in each dish with a little of the chilli pepper, spring onions and abalone, if using. Break an egg into each bowl and season with soy sauce, salt and pepper. Stand the ramekins on a baking sheet and bake in a preheated oven at 200¬∞ C/400¬∞ F/gas mark 6 for about 15 minutes until the eggs are set and slightly crisp around the outside. Lift them carefully on to a warmed serving plate and garnish with parsley.

Prawn Egg Rolls

Serves 4

225 g/8 oz bean sprouts
30 ml/2 tbsp groundnut (peanut) oil
4 stalks celery, chopped
100 g/4 oz mushrooms, chopped
225 g/8 oz peeled prawns, chopped
15 ml/1 tbsp rice wine or dry sherry
2.5 ml/¬Ω tsp cornflour (cornstarch)
2.5 ml/¬Ω tsp salt
2.5 ml/¬Ω tsp sugar
12 egg roll skins
1 egg, beaten
oil for deep-frying

Blanch the bean sprouts in boiling water for 2 minutes then drain. Heat the oil and stir-fry the celery for 1 minute. Add the mushrooms and stir-fry for 1 minute. Add the prawns, wine or sherry, cornflour, salt and sugar and stir-fry for 2 minutes. Leave to cool.

Place a little of the filling on the centre of each skin and brush the edges with beaten egg. Fold in the edges then roll the egg roll away from you, sealing the edges with egg. Heat the oil and deep-fry until golden brown.

Far Eastern Style Prawns

Serves 4

16,Äì20 peeled king prawns

juice of 1 lemon

120 ml/4 fl oz/¬Ω cup dry white wine

30 ml/2 tbsp soy sauce

30 ml/2 tbsp honey

15 ml/1 tbsp grated lemon rind

salt and pepper

45 ml/3 tbsp groundnut (peanut) oil

1 clove garlic, chopped

6 spring onions (scallions), cut into strips

2 carrots, cut into strips

5 ml/1 tsp five-spice powder

5 ml/1 tsp cornflour (cornstarch)

Mix the prawns with the lemon juice, wine, soy sauce, honey and lemon rind and season with salt and pepper. Cover and marinate for 1 hour. Heat the oil and fry the garlic until lightly browned. Add the vegetables and stir-fry until tender but still crisp. Drain the prawns, add them to the pan and stir-fry for 2 minutes. Strain the marinade and mix it with the five-spice powder and cornflour. Add to the wok, stir well and bring to the boil.

Prawn Foo Yung

Serves 4

6 eggs, beaten

45 ml/3 tbsp cornflour (cornstarch)

225 g/8 oz peeled prawns

100 g/4 oz mushrooms, sliced

5 ml/1 tsp salt

2 spring onions (scallions), chopped

45 ml/3 tbsp groundnut (peanut) oil

Beat the eggs then beat in the cornflour. Add all the remaining ingredients except the oil. Heat the oil and pour the mixture into the pan a little at a time to make pancakes about 7.5 cm/3 in across. Fry until the bottom is golden brown then turn and brown the other side.

Prawn Fries

Serves 4

12 large uncooked prawns
1 egg, beaten
30 ml/2 tbsp cornflour (cornstarch)
pinch of salt
pinch of pepper
3 slices bread
1 hard-boiled (hard-cooked) egg yolk, chopped
25 g/1 oz cooked ham, chopped
1 spring onion (scallion), chopped
oil for deep-frying

Remove the shells and back veins from the prawns, leaving the tails intact. Cut down the back of the prawns with a sharp knife and gently press them flat. Beat the egg, cornflour, salt and pepper. Toss the prawns in the mixture until completely coated. Remove the crusts from the bread and cut it into quarters. Place one prawn, cut side down, on each piece and press down. Brush a little egg mixture over each prawn then sprinkle with the egg yolk, ham and spring onion. Heat the oil and fry the prawn bread pieces in batches until golden. Drain on kitchen paper and serve hot.

Fried Prawns in Sauce

Serves 4

75 g/3 oz/heaped ¬° cup cornflour (cornstarch)

¬Ω egg, beaten

5 ml/1 tsp rice wine or dry sherry

salt

450 g/1 lb peeled prawns

45 ml/3 tbsp groundnut (peanut) oil

5 ml/1 tsp sesame oil

1 clove garlic, crushed

1 slice ginger root, minced

3 spring onions (scallions), sliced

15 ml/1 tbsp fish stock

5 ml/1 tsp wine vinegar

5 ml/1 tsp sugar

Mix together the cornflour, egg, wine or sherry and a pinch of salt to make a batter. Dip the prawns in the batter so that they are lightly coated. Heat the oil and fry the prawns until they are crisp outside. Remove them from the pan and drain off the oil. Heat the sesame oil in the pan, add the prawns, garlic, ginger and spring onions and stir-fry for 3 minutes. Stir in the stock, wine vinegar and sugar, stir well and heat through before serving.

Poached Prawns with Ham and Tofu

Serves 4

30 ml/2 tbsp groundnut (peanut) oil

225 g/8 oz tofu, cubed

600 ml/1 pt/2¬Ω cups chicken stock

100 g/4 oz smoked ham, cubed

225 g/8 oz peeled prawns

Heat the oil and fry the tofu until lightly browned. Remove from the pan and drain. Heat the stock, add the tofu and ham and simmer gently for about 10 minutes until the tofu is cooked. Add the prawns and simmer for a further 5 minutes until heated through. Serve in deep bowls.

Prawns in Lobster Sauce

Serves 4

45 ml/3 tbsp groundnut (peanut) oil

2 cloves garlic, crushed

5 ml/1 tsp minced black beans

100 g/4 oz minced (ground) pork

450 g/1 lb peeled prawns

15 ml/1 tbsp rice wine or dry sherry

300 ml/¬Ω pt/1¬° cups chicken stock

30 ml/2 tbsp cornflour (cornstarch)

2 eggs, beaten

15 ml/1 tbsp soy sauce

2.5 ml/¬Ω tsp salt

2.5 ml/¬Ω tsp sugar

2 spring onions (scallions), chopped

Heat the oil and fry the garlic and black beans until the garlic is
until lightly browned. Add the pork and fry until browned. Add
the prawns and stir-fry for 1 minute. Add the sherry, cover and
simmer for 1 minute. Add the stock and cornflour, bring to the
boil, stirring, cover and simmer for 5 minutes. Add the eggs,
stirring all the time so that they form into threads. Add the soy

sauce, salt, sugar and spring onions and simmer for a few minutes before serving.

Ingram Content Group UK Ltd.
Milton Keynes UK
UKHW021103310323
419467UK00015B/497

9 781802 909586